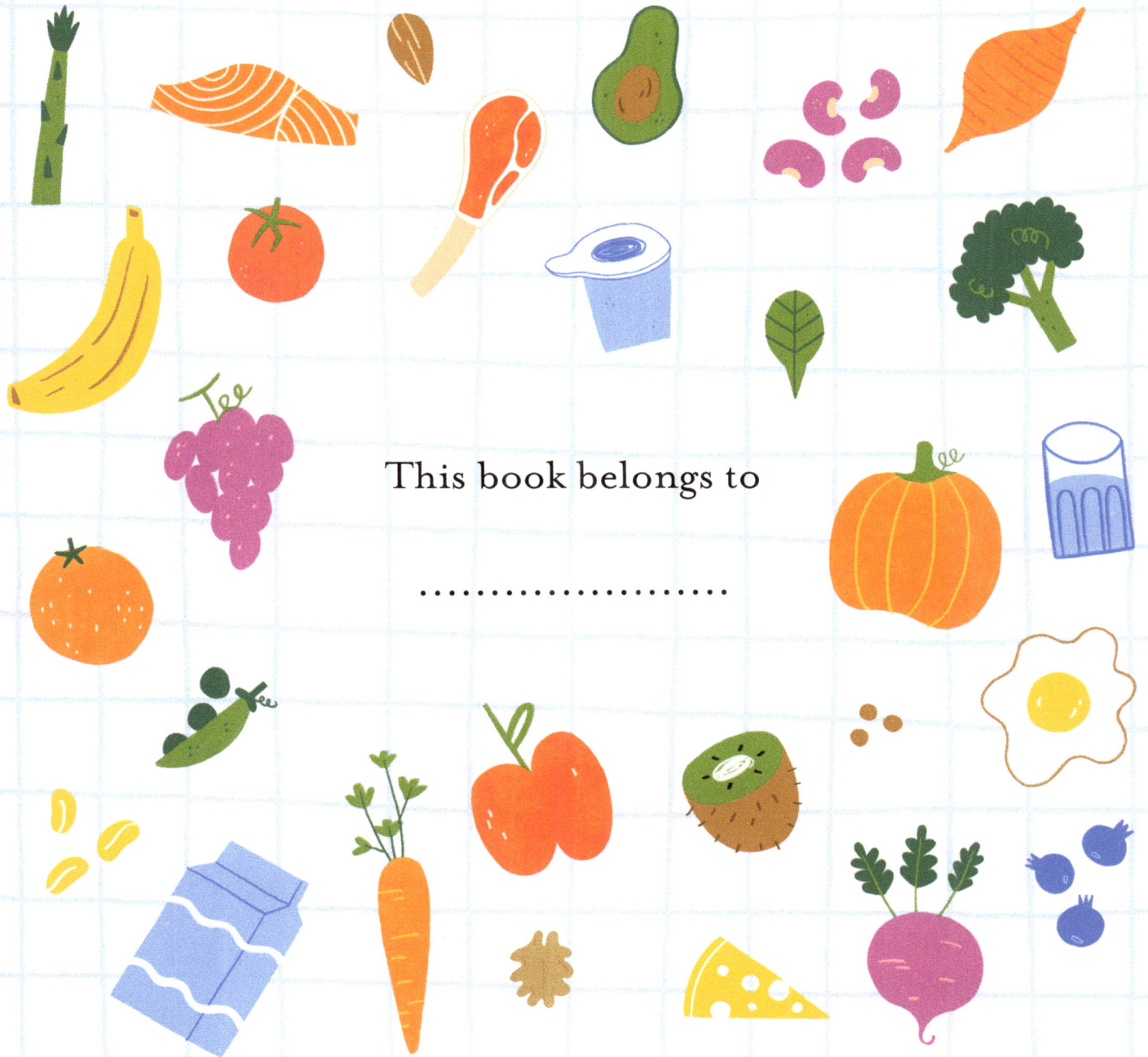

This book belongs to

....

For Heidi, Josie, Leni,
and those still to come.
Our bodies and food
can be so much fun!

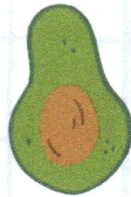

What Does All My Food Do?
Written by Shell Stewart
Illustrated by Claudia Fasser
Copyright © 2024 by Shell Stewart
All rights reserved.
No part of this book may be reproduced in
any manner whatsoever without prior written
permission of the publisher.
First Printing, 2024
Published by Newport Road Press
www.newportroadpress.com.au
ABN 65419524367
ISBN 978-1-7635313-0-7 Hardcover version
ISBN 978-1-7635313-1-4 Paperback version

WHAT DOES ALL MY FOOD DO?

Written by Shell Stewart
Illustrated by Claudia Fasser

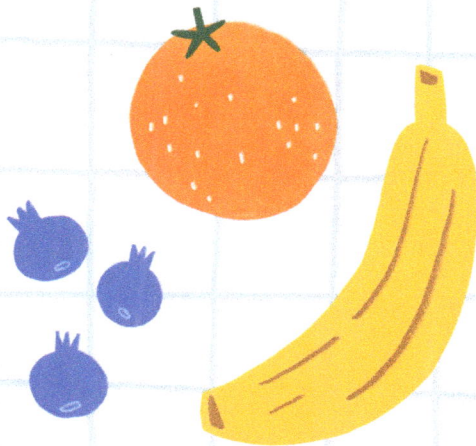

What does all my food do
when I chew and chew and chew?

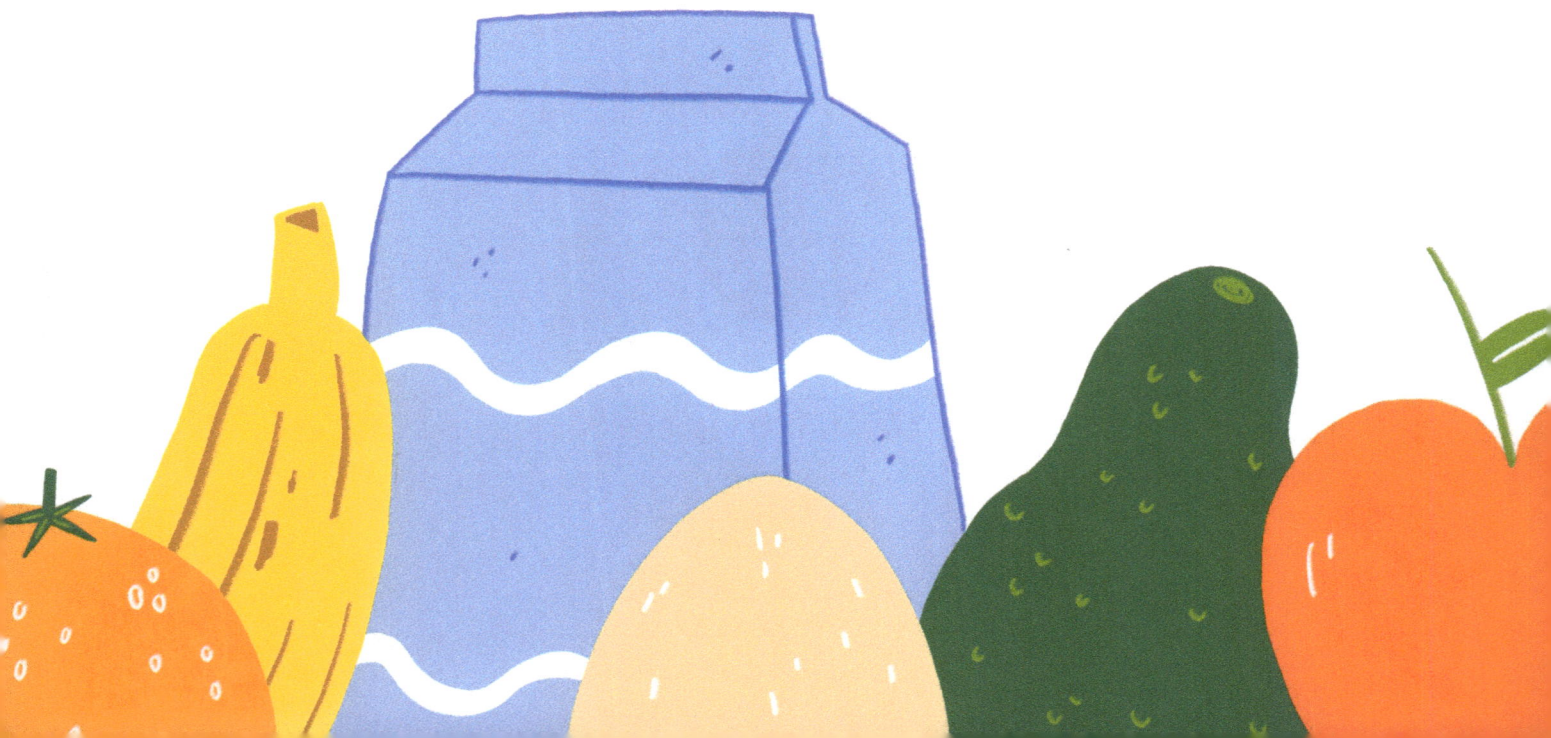

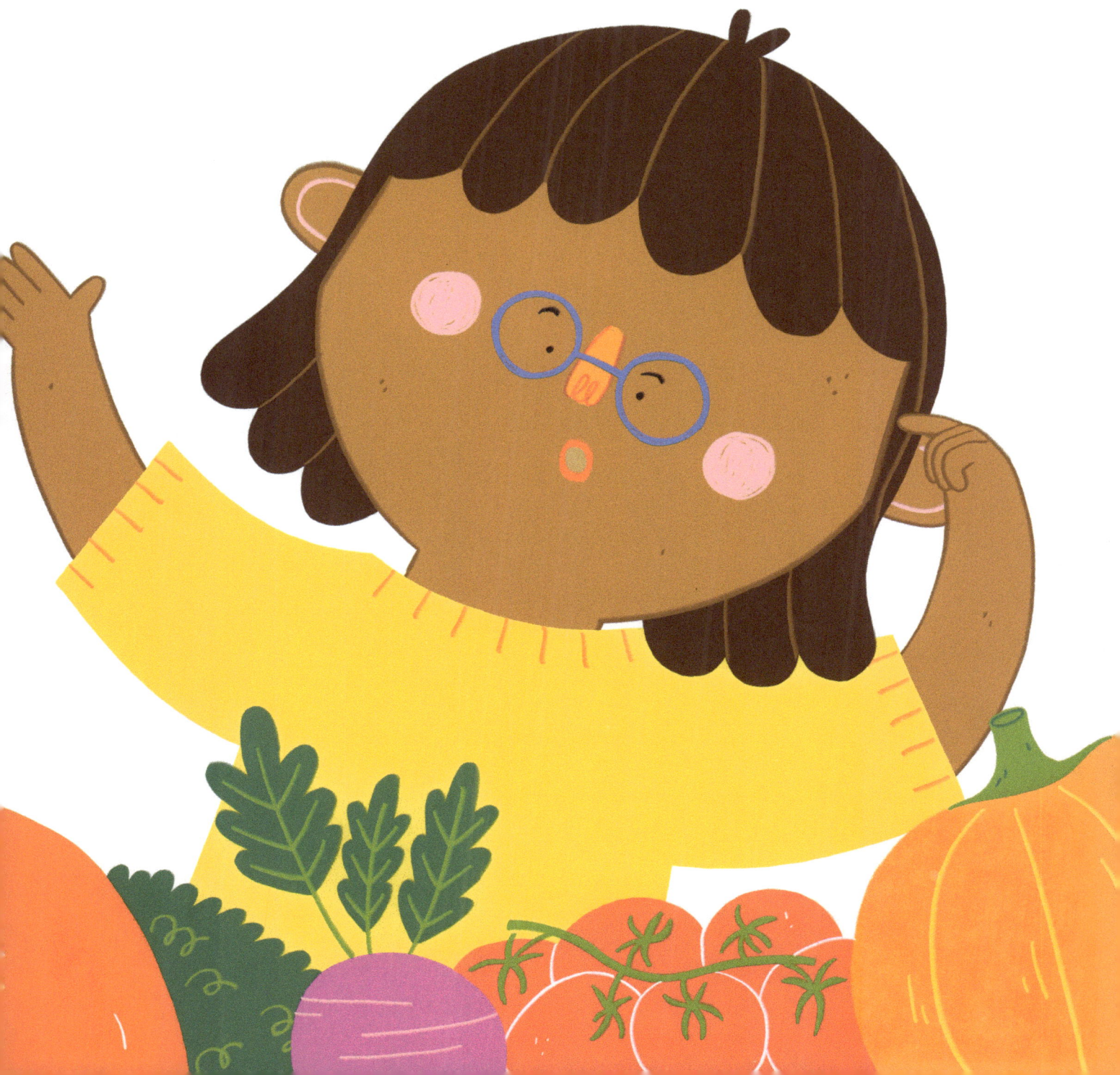

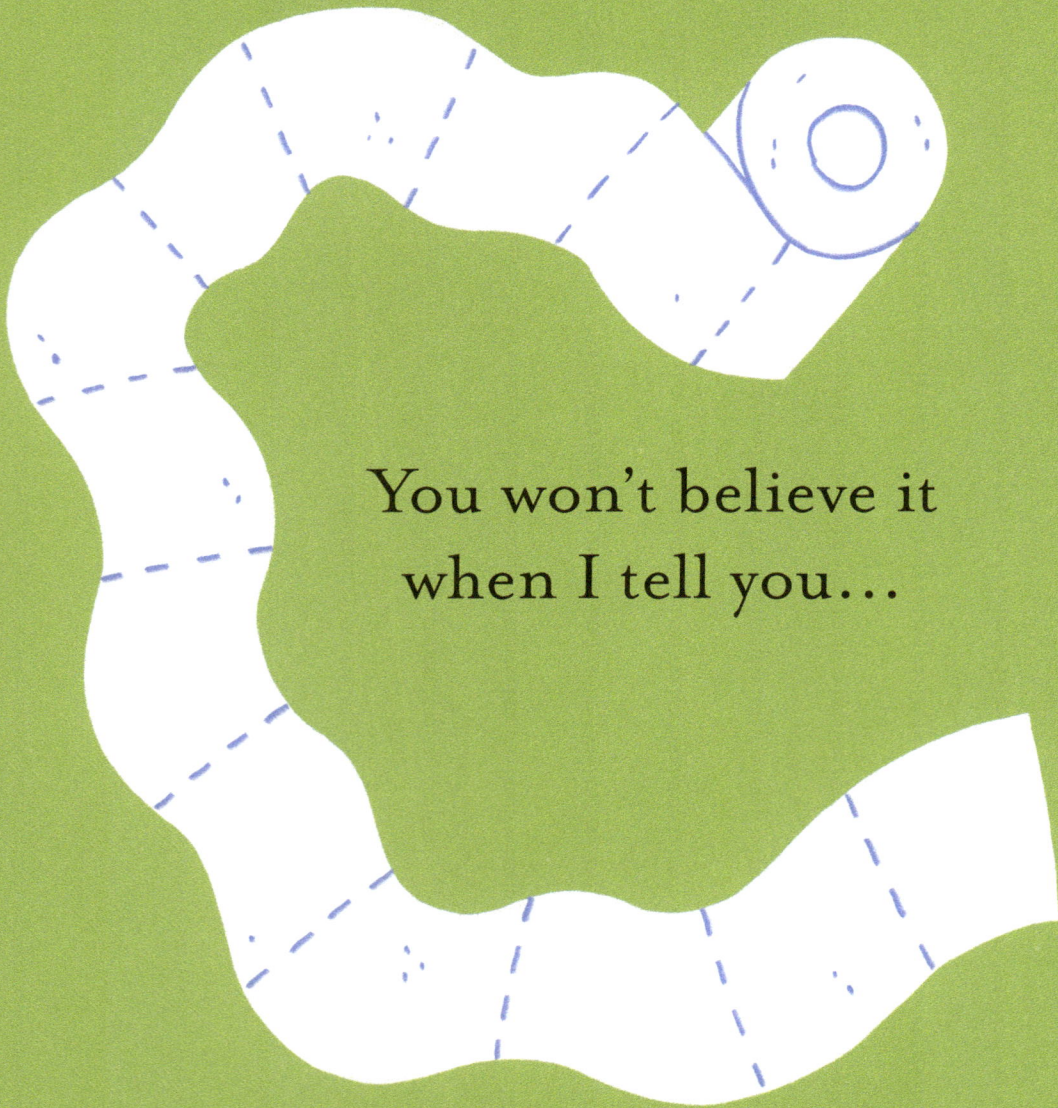

You won't believe it
when I tell you…

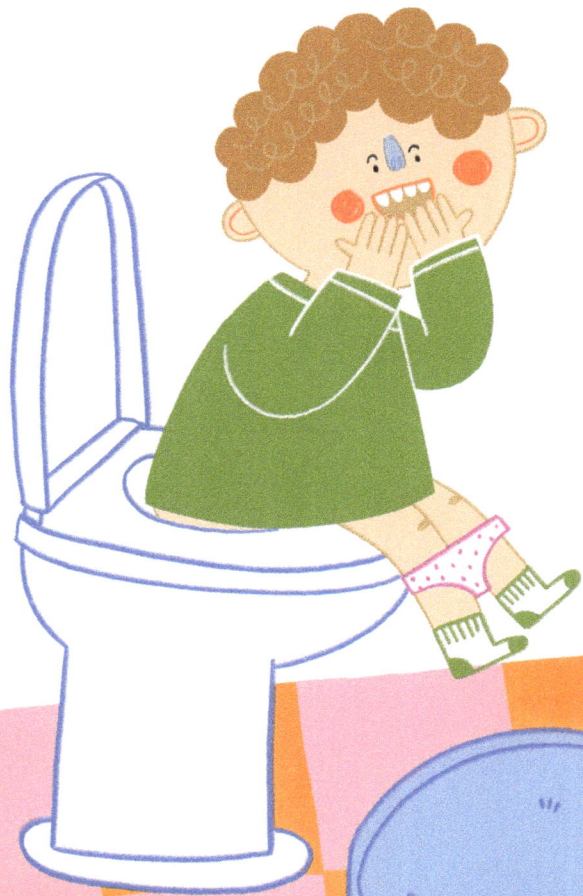

it comes out as... POO.

But before our food turns brown,
it has important jobs to do.

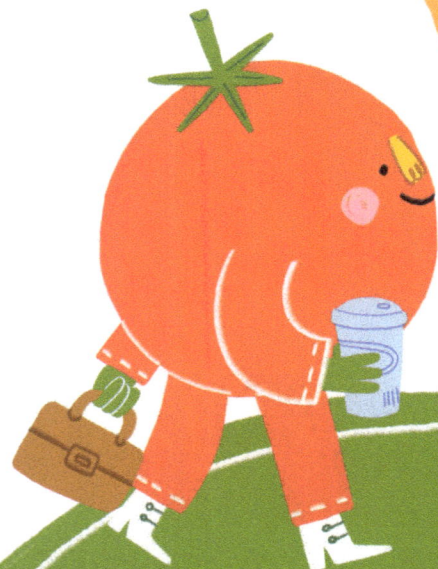

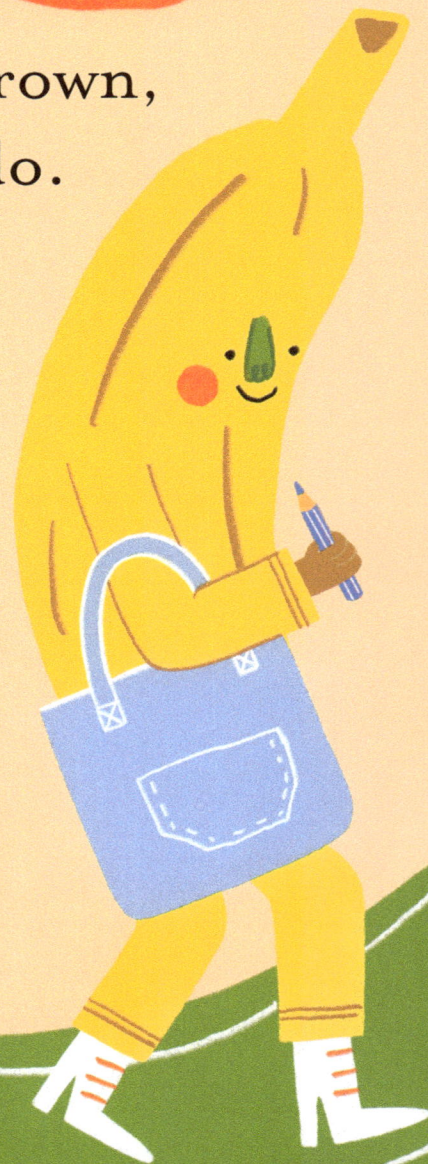

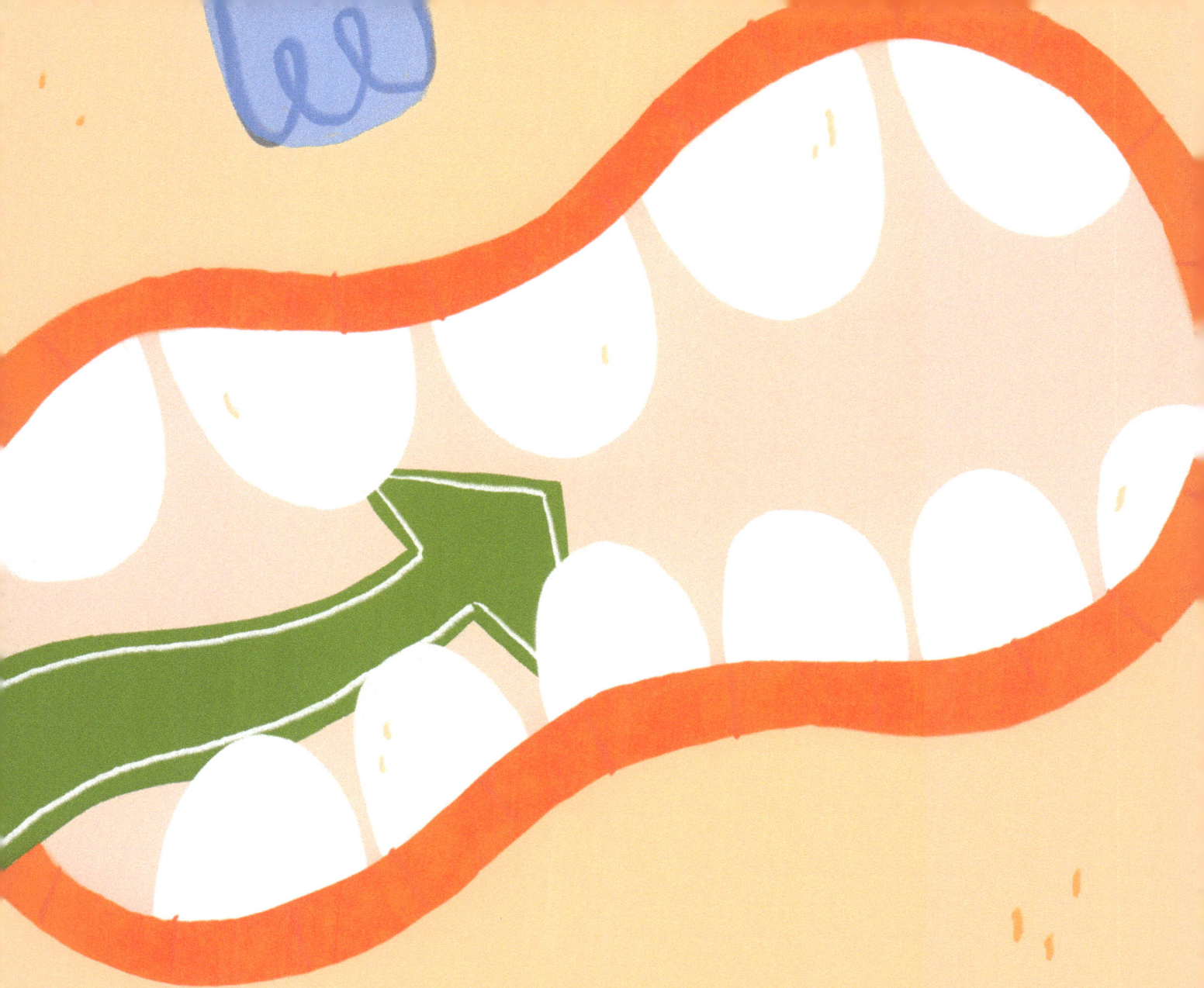

Our yummy food gets straight to work
inside me and you!

My oats, salmon and spinach
go down into my tummy.

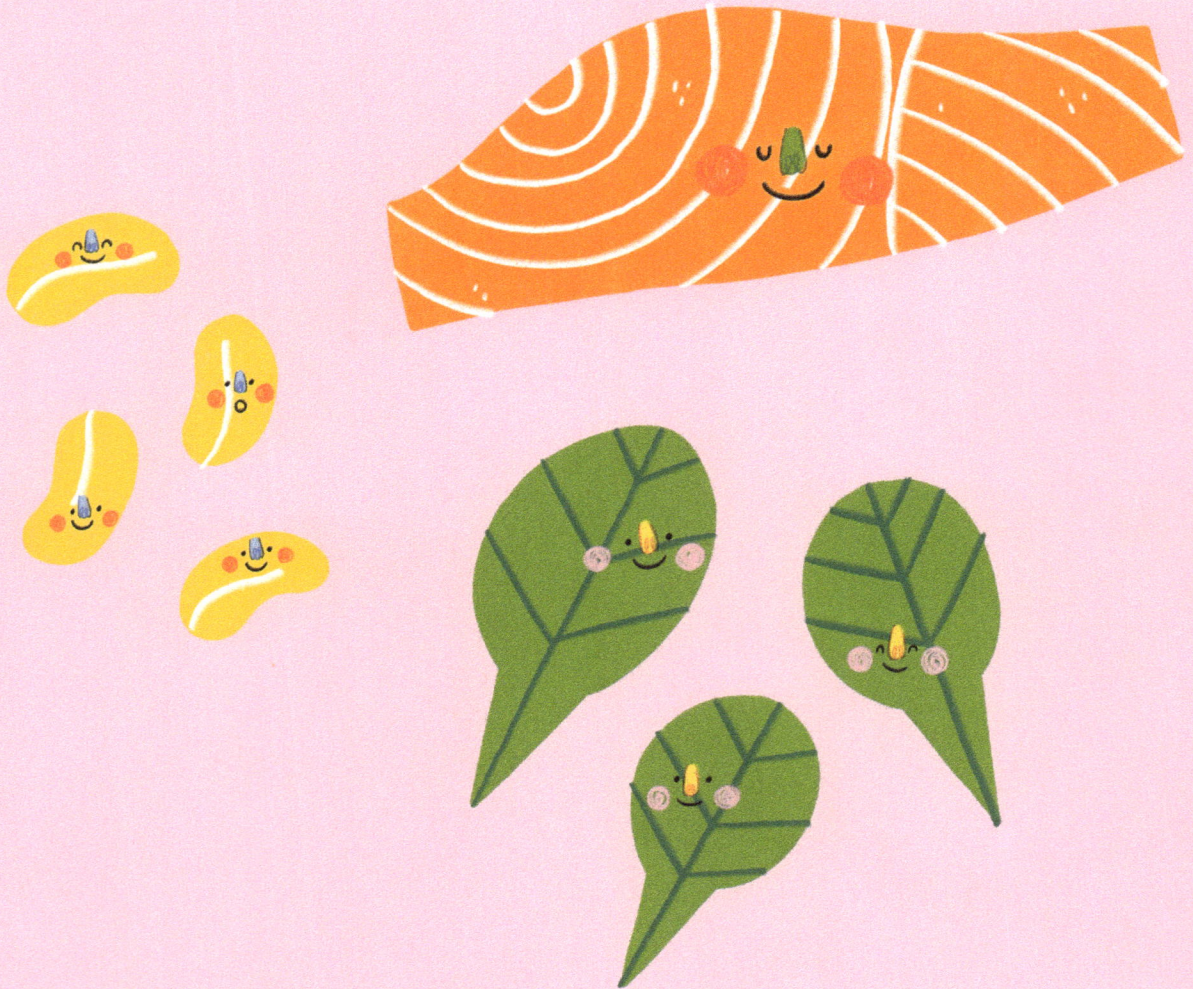

Then what do they do?

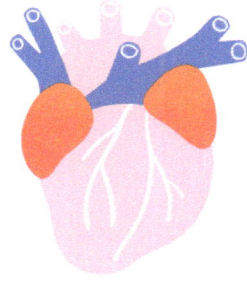

They help my HEART to beat strong
so I can play all day long.

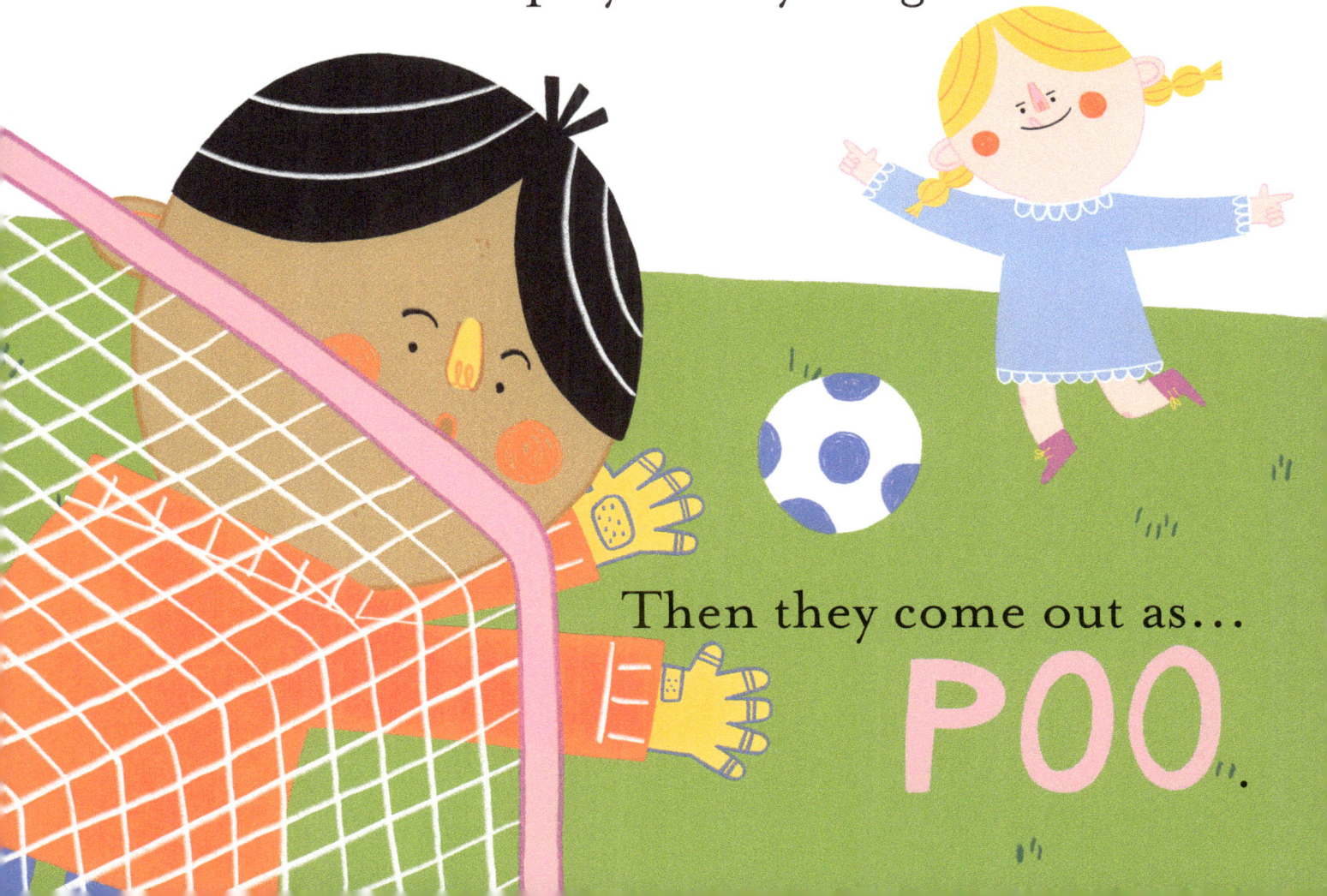

Then they come out as...

POO.

My blueberries, nuts and avocado
go down into my tummy.

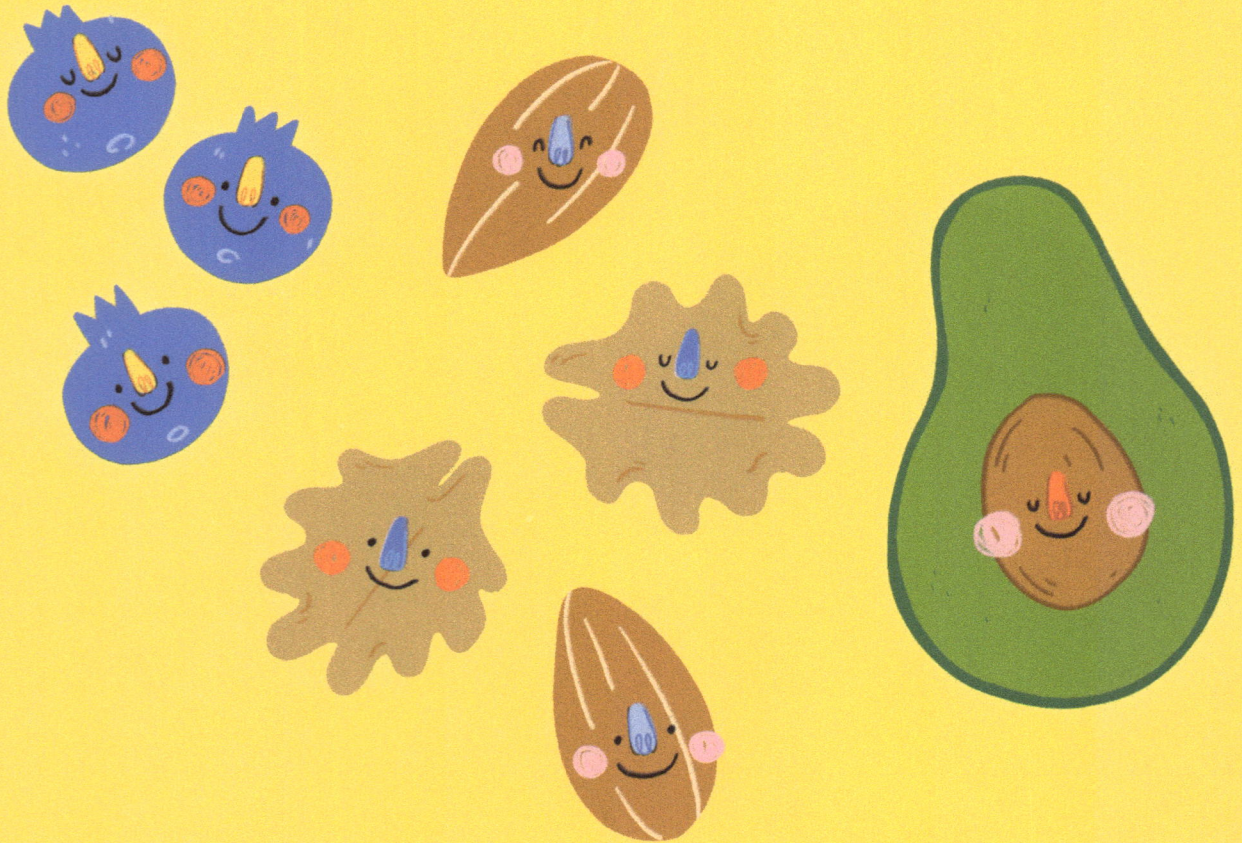

Then what do they do?

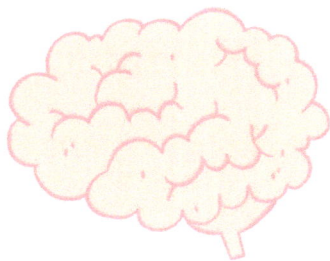

They help my BRAIN to be clever
so I can learn cool things forever.

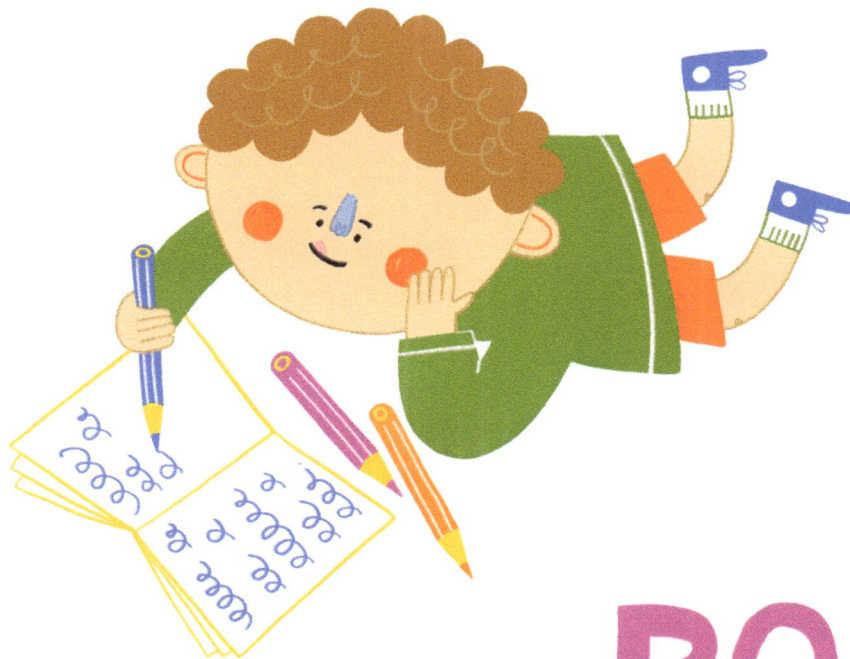

Then they come out as... POO.

My beetroot, pumpkin and lentils
go down into my tummy.

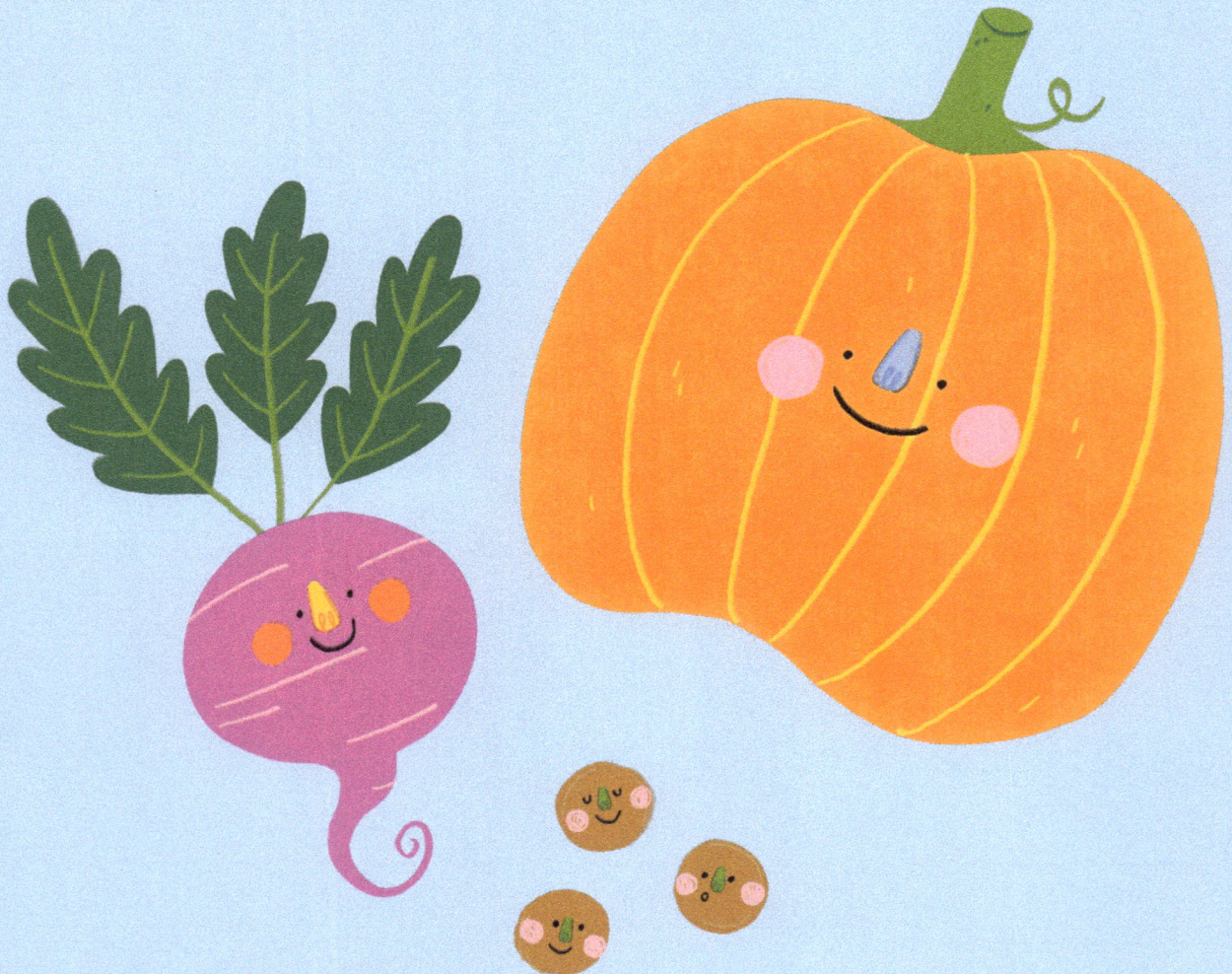

Then what do they do?

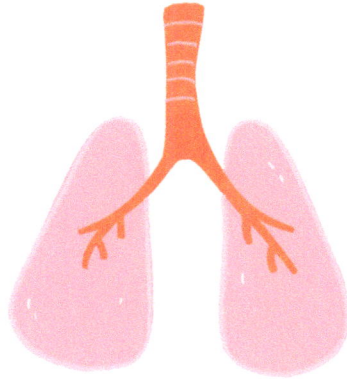

They help my LUNGS to fill with air
so I can sing without a care.

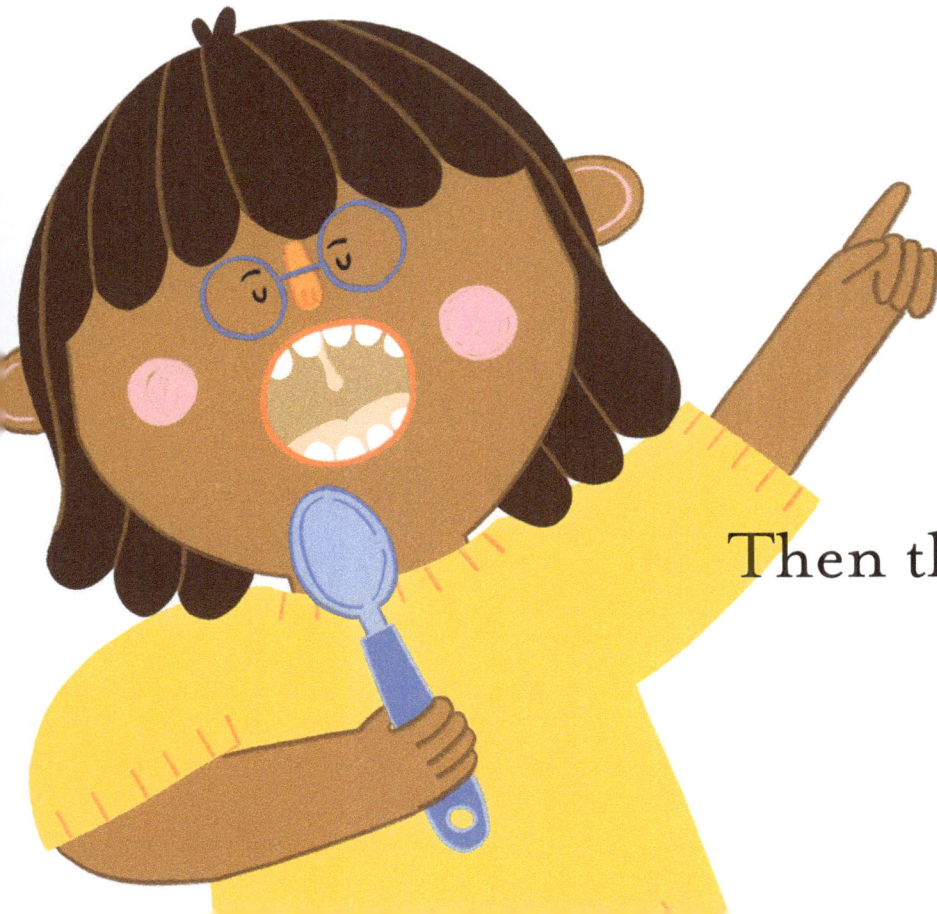

Then they come out as...

POO.

My cheese, milk and broccoli
go down into my tummy.

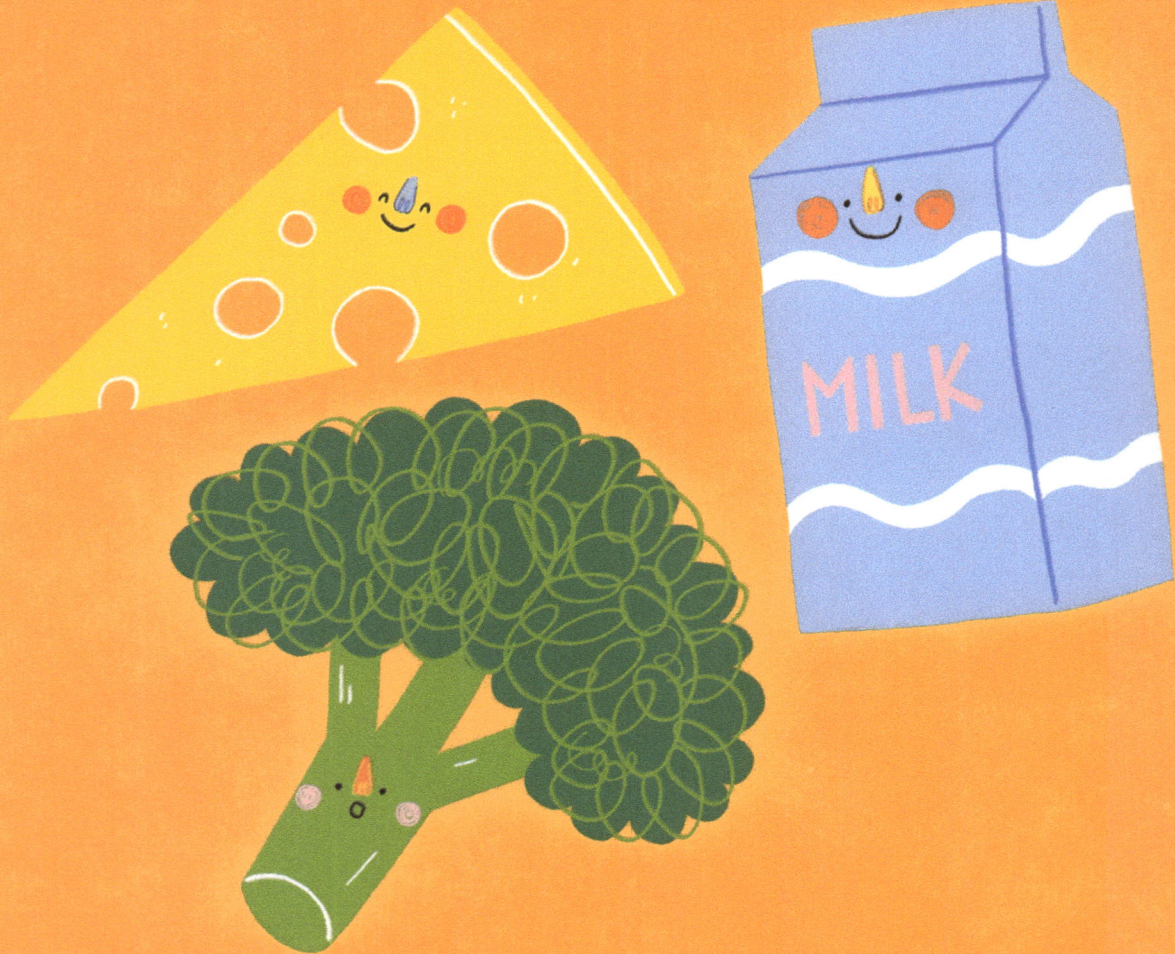

Then what do they do?

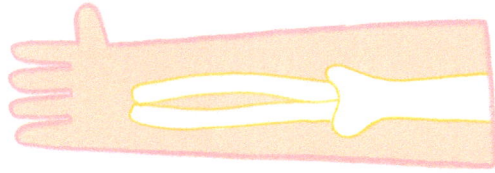

They help my BONES to grow strong and hard so I can play in my backyard.

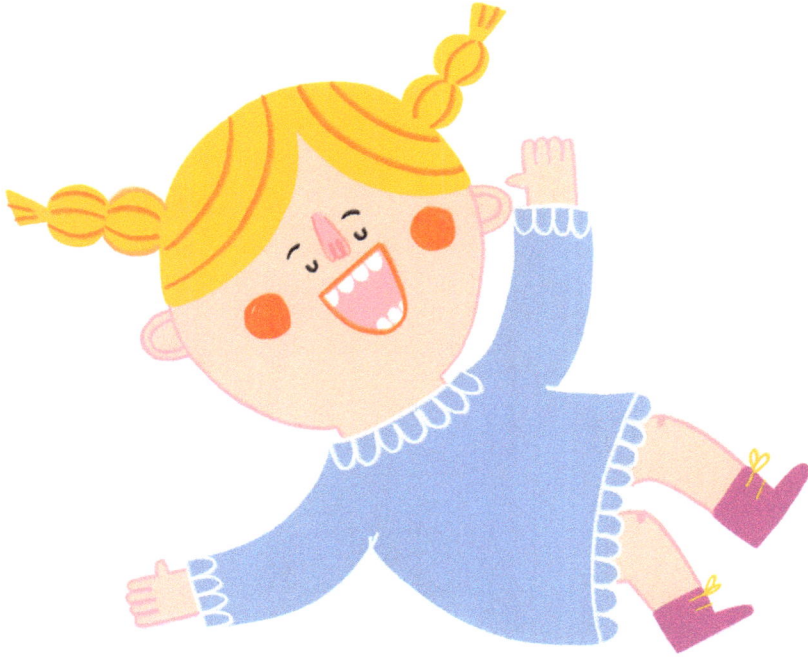

Then they come out as... **POO**.

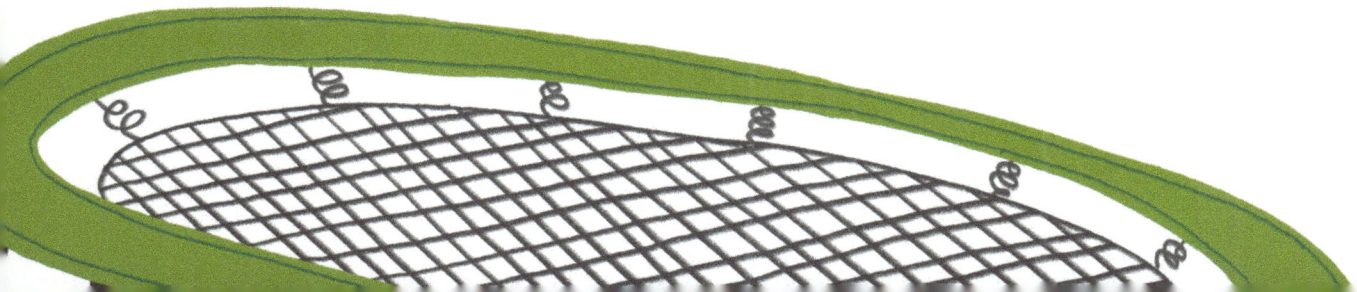

My egg, meat and beans
go down into my tummy.

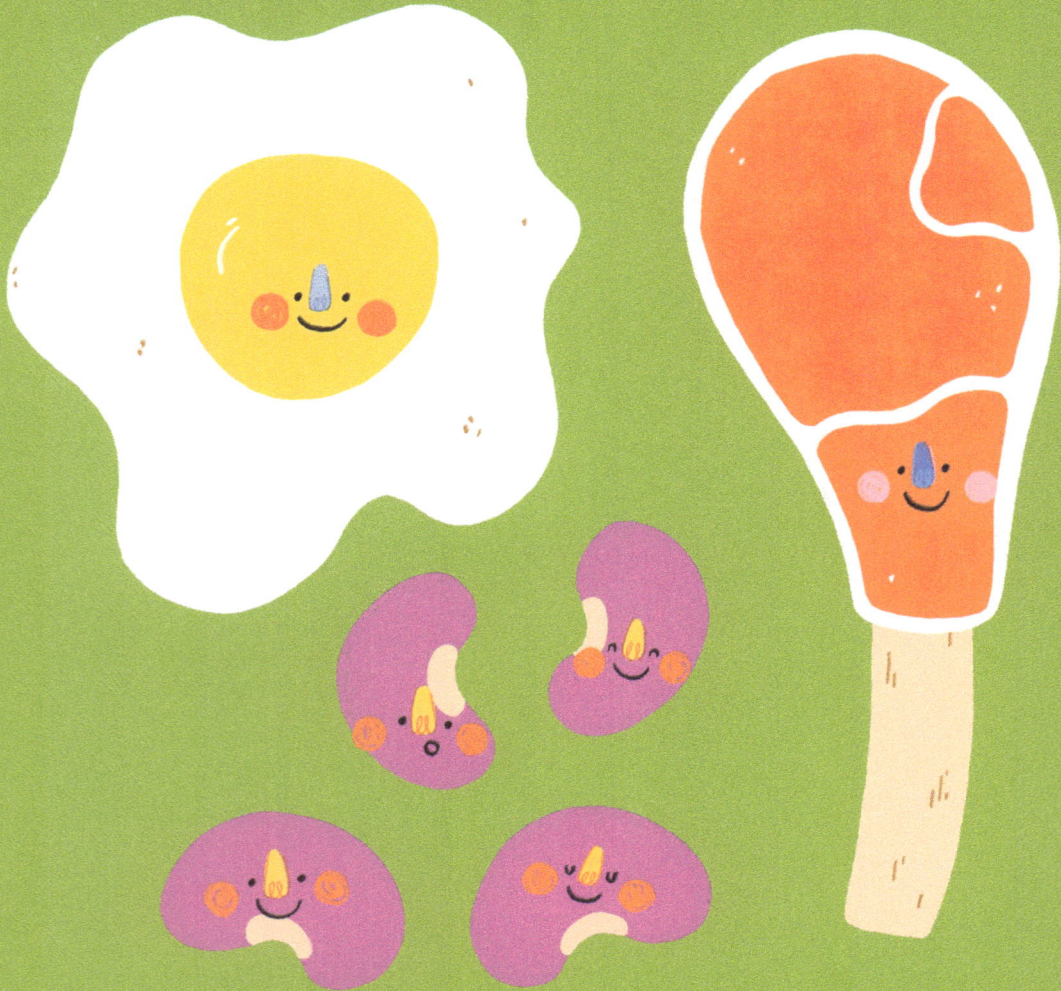

Then what do they do?

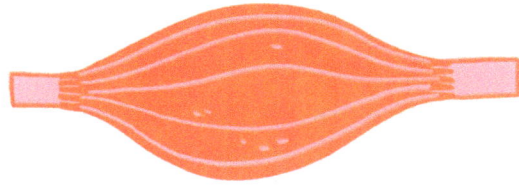

They help my MUSCLES get me moving
so I can keep on grooving.

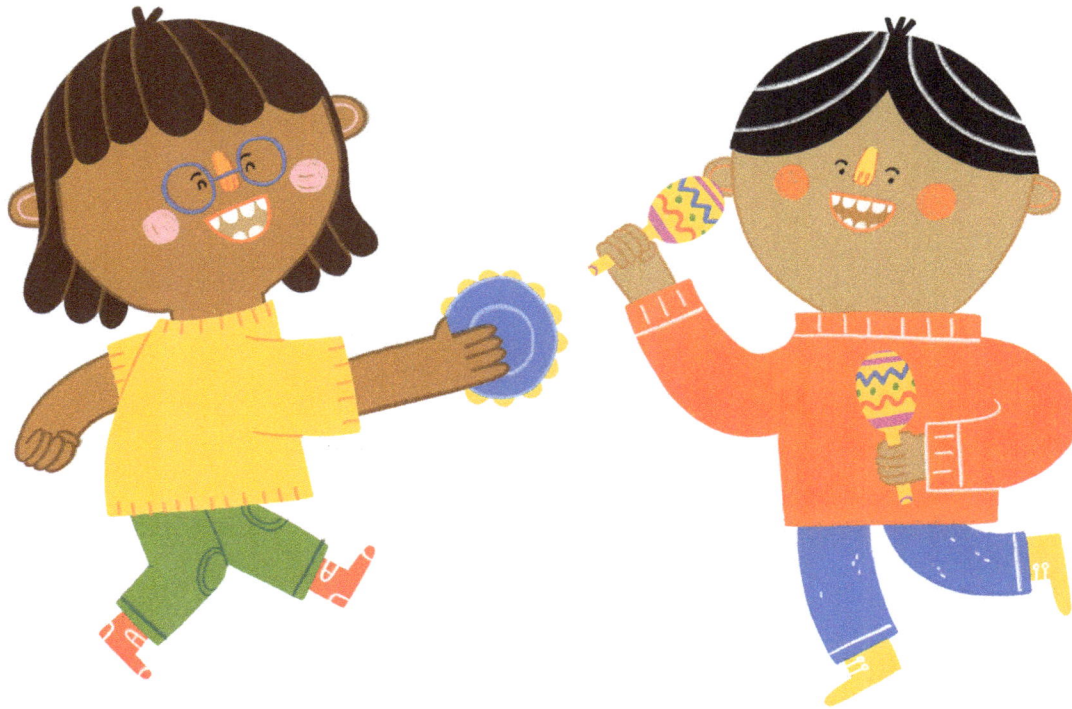

Then they come out as…

POO.

My carrot, peas and orange
go down into my tummy.

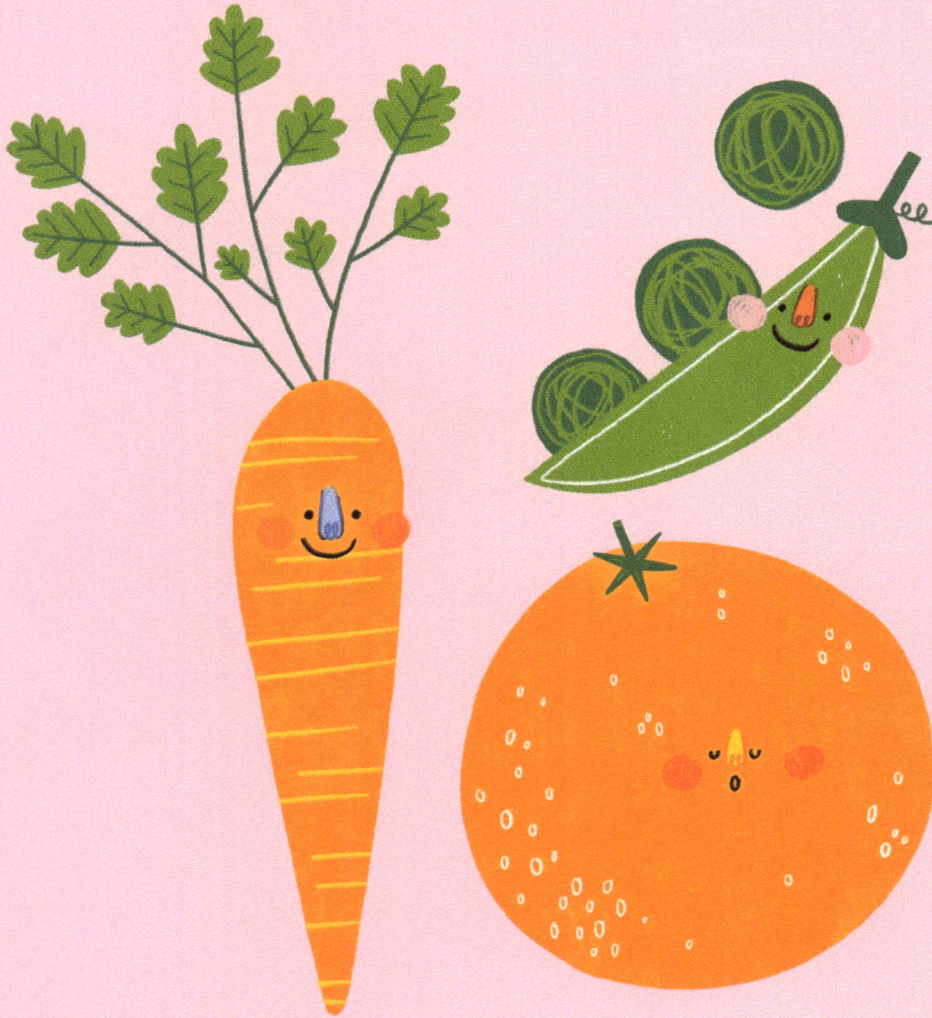

Then what do they do?

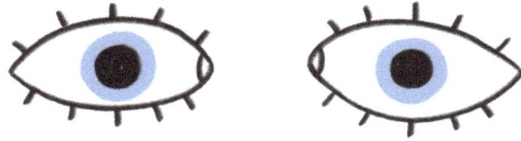

They help my EYES to open wide
so I can see the world outside.

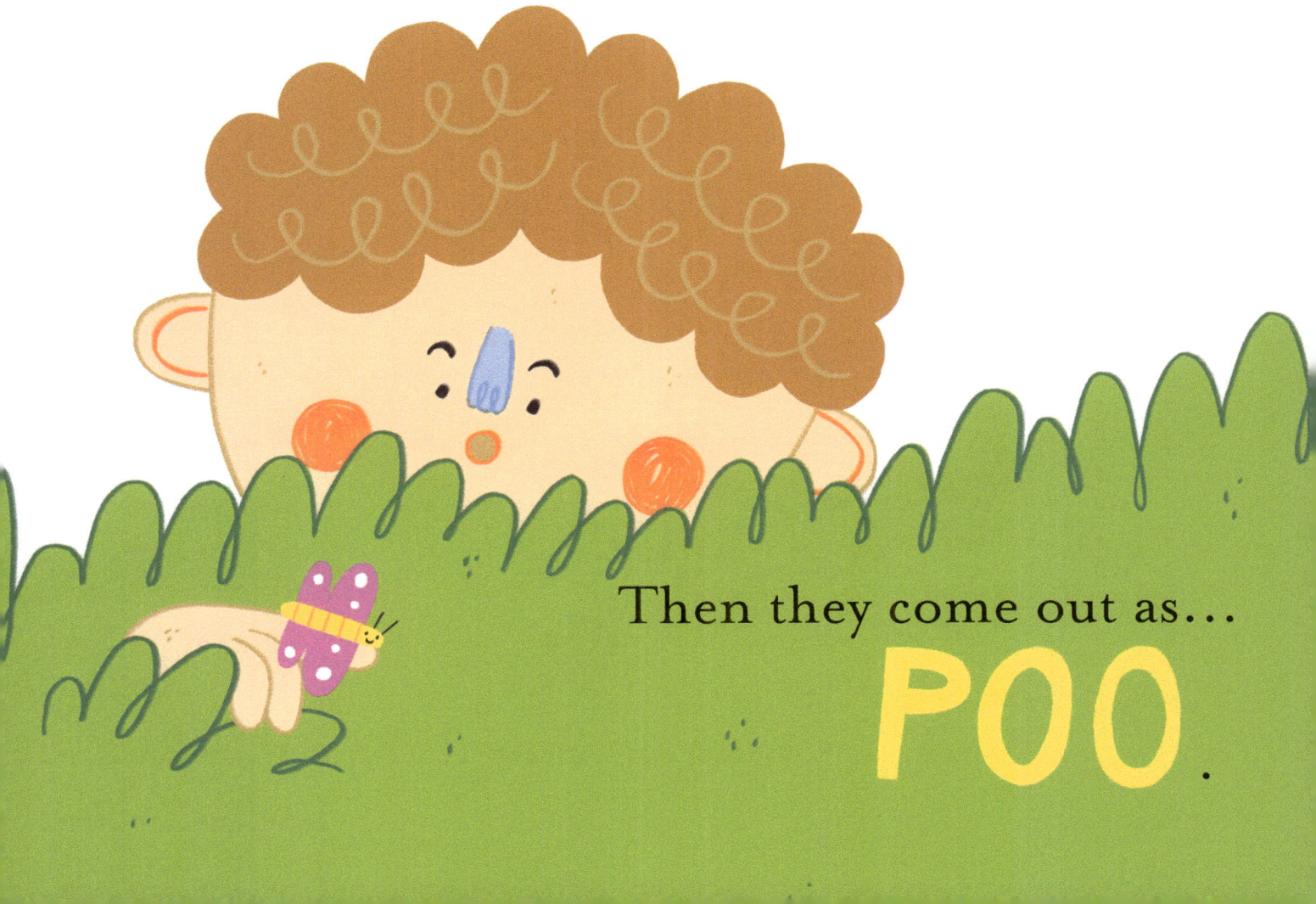

Then they come out as...
POO.

My tomato, grapes and sweet potato
go down into my tummy.

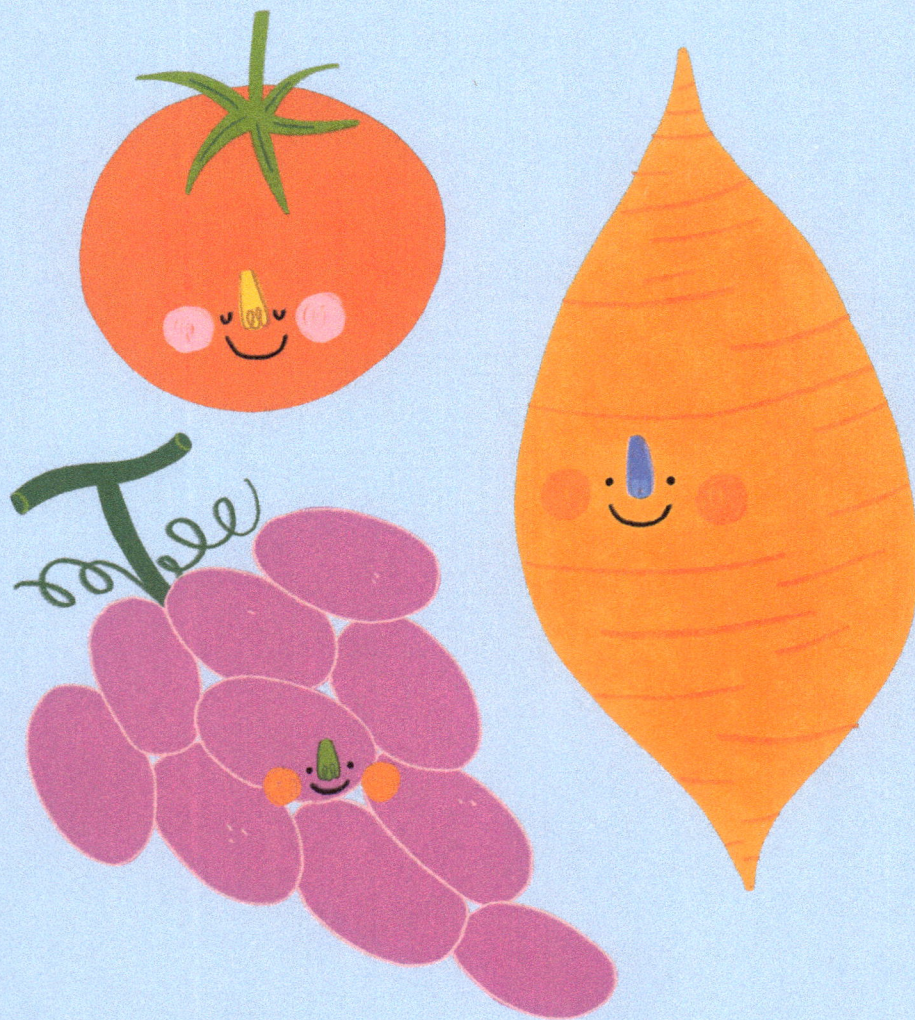

Then what do they do?

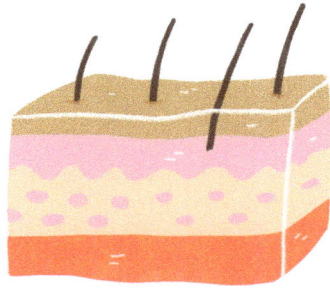

They help my SKIN to mend and heal
if I fall off my set of wheels.

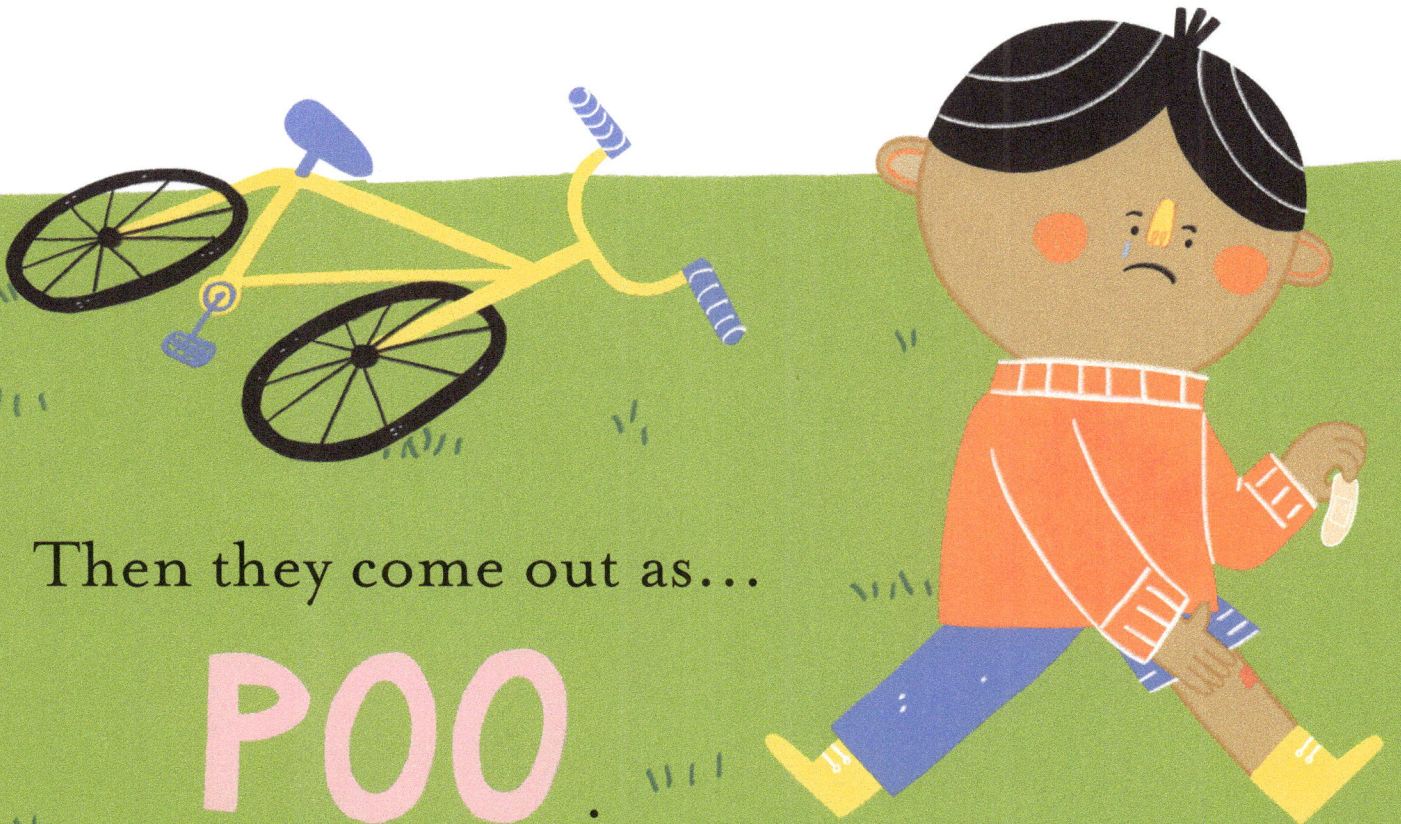

Then they come out as...

POO.

My apple, water and kiwi fruit
go down into my tummy.

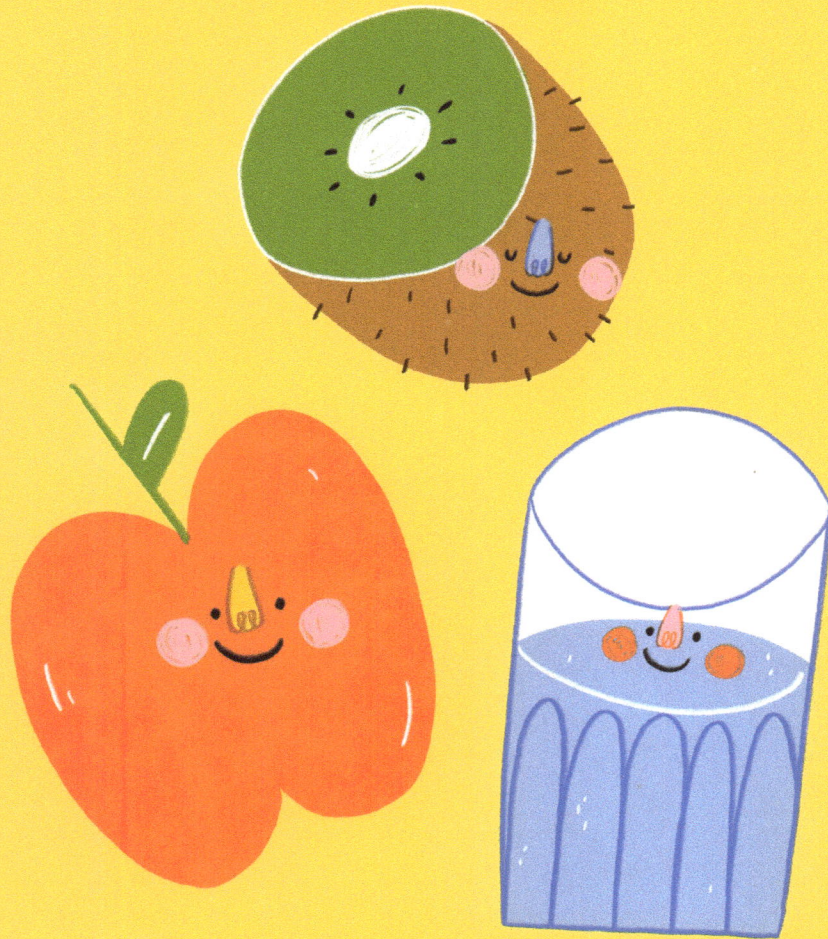

Then what do they do?

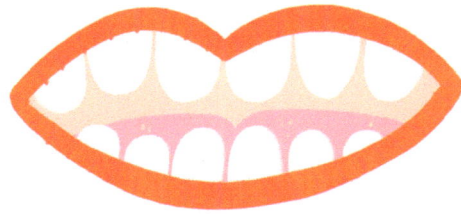

They help my TEETH stay strong and white
so I can chew and smile so bright.

Then they come out as…

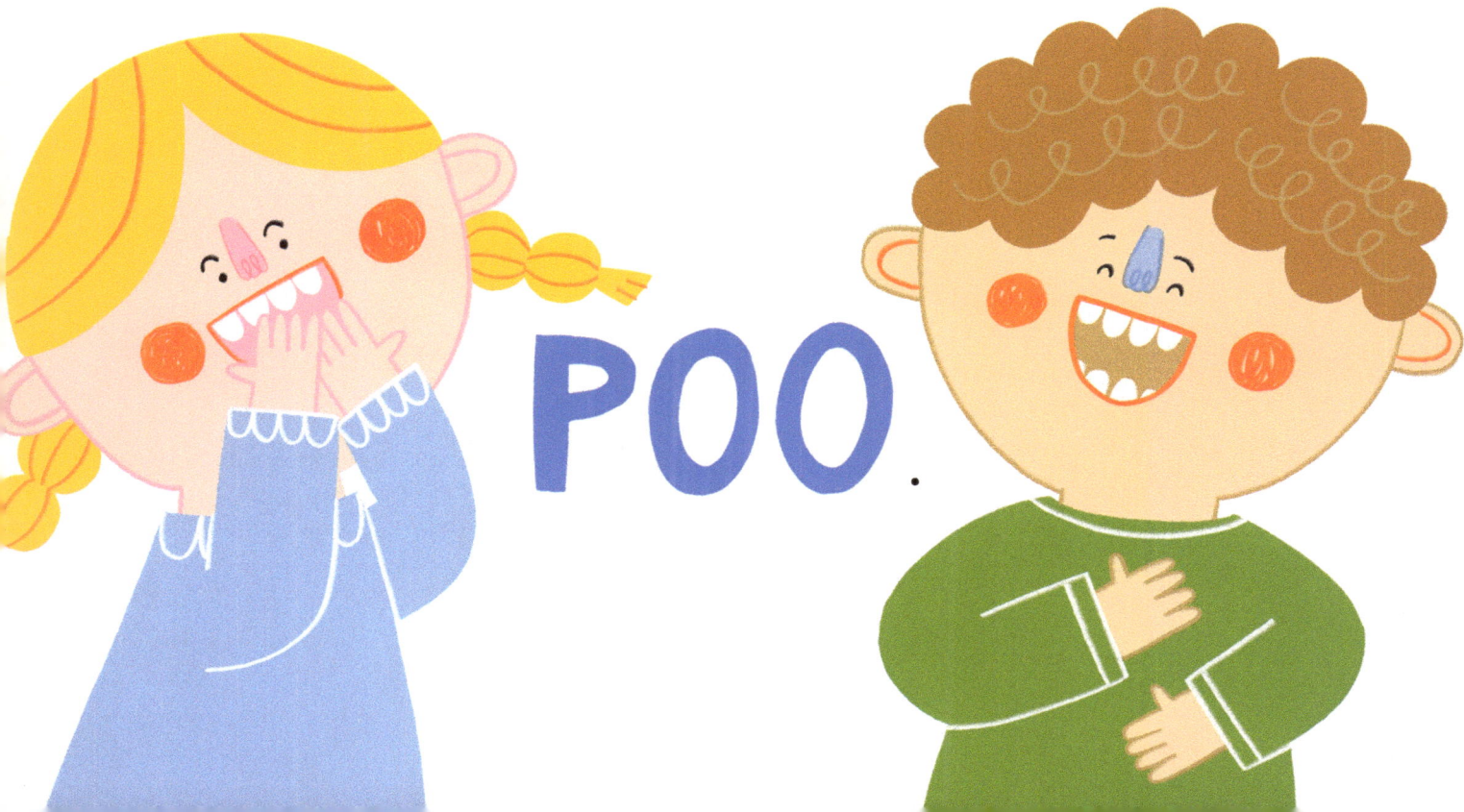

POO.

My yogurt, asparagus and banana
go down into my tummy.

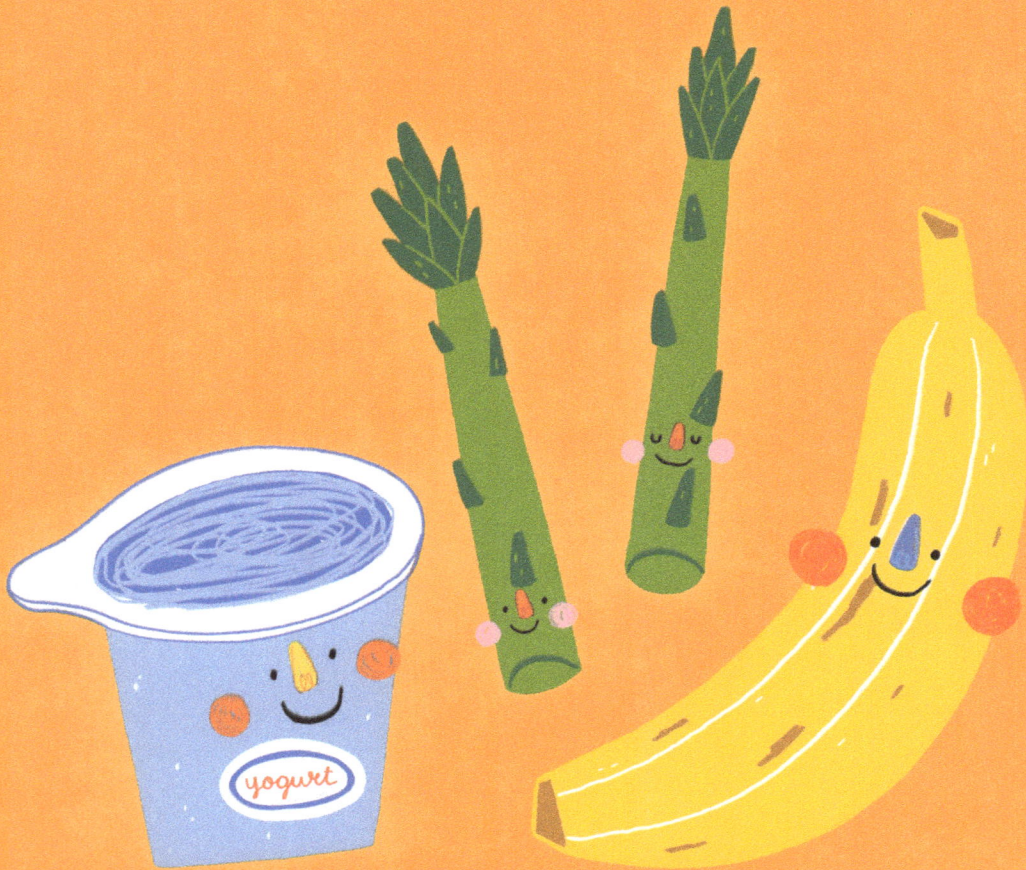

Then what do they do?

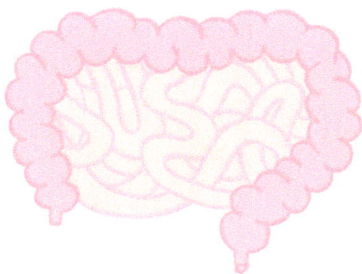

They help my INTESTINES digest food that I have bitten, munched and chewed.

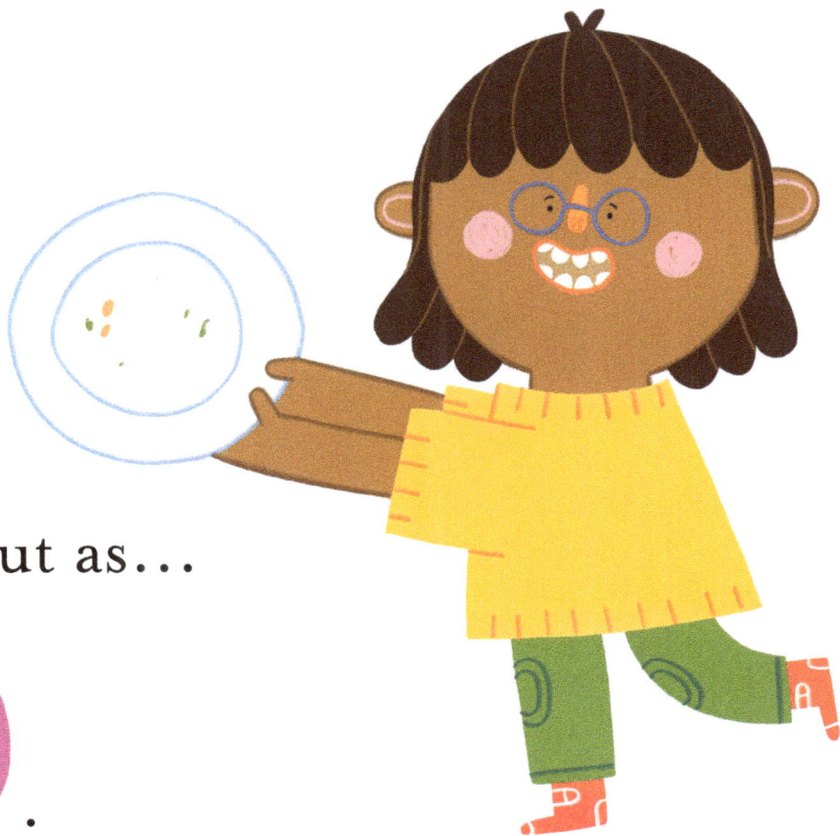

Then they come out as...

POO.

So when you swallow something yummy
down into your tummy…

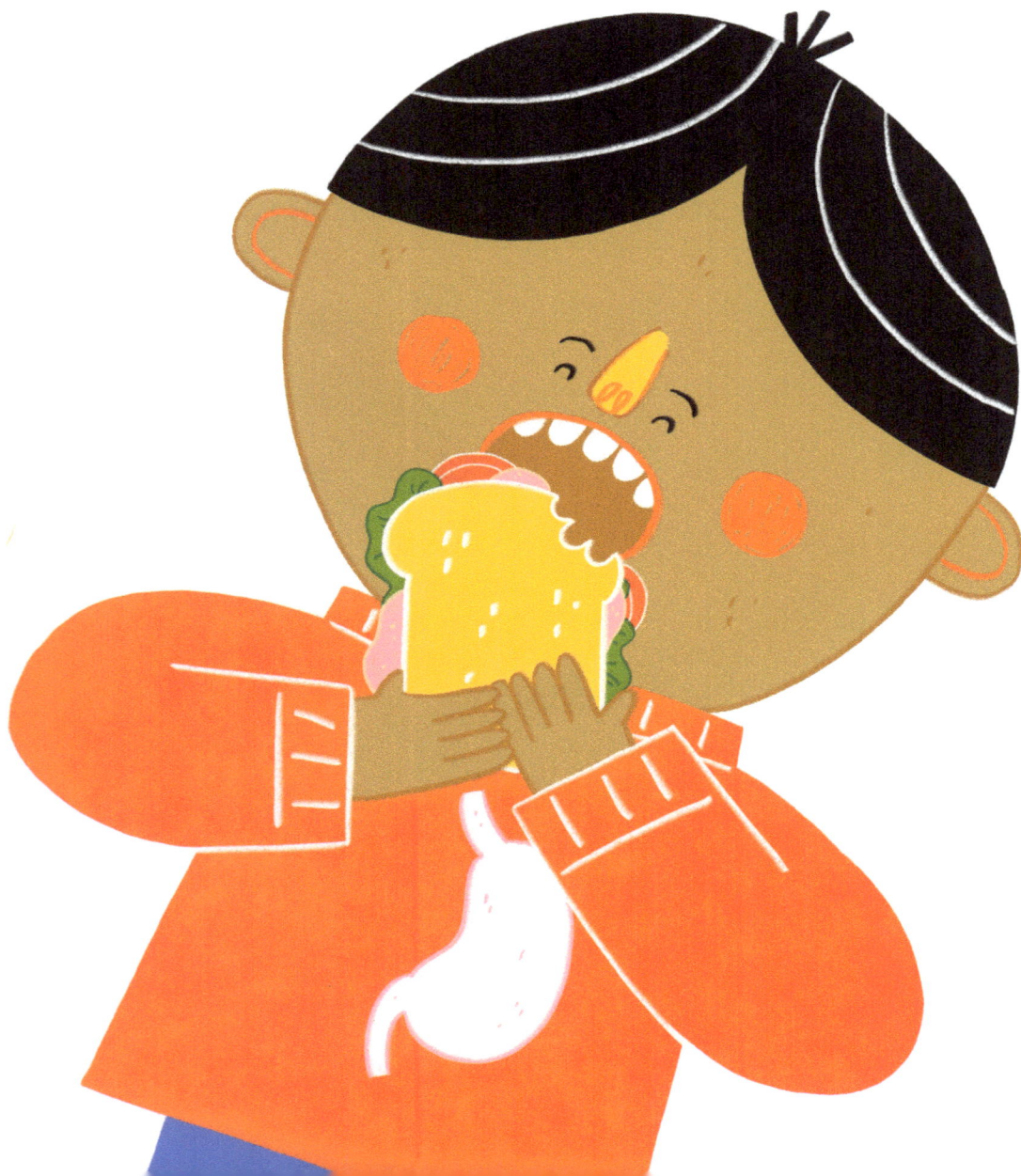

Remember your food works hard for you,

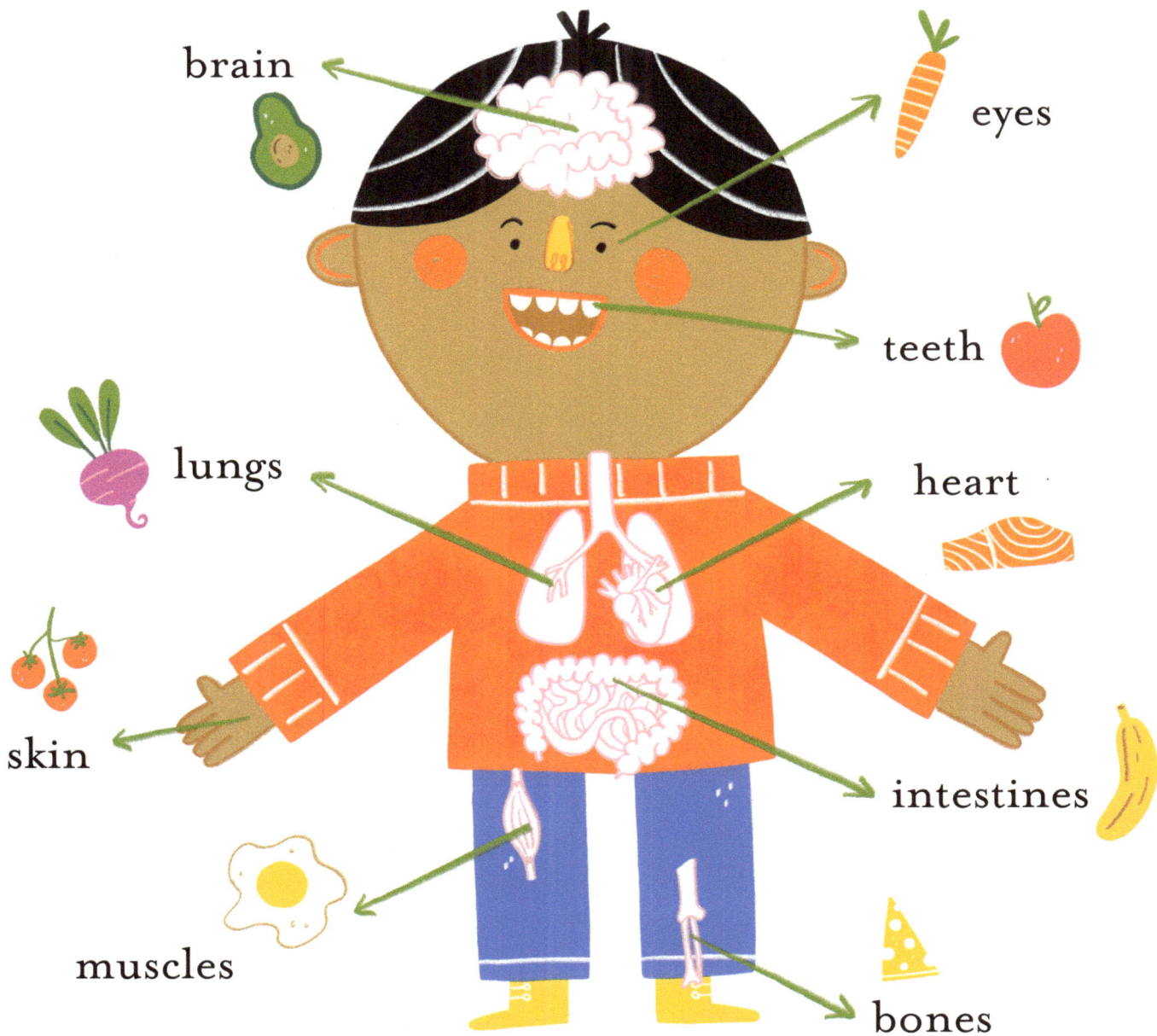

brain

eyes

teeth

lungs

heart

skin

intestines

muscles

bones

before it comes out as…

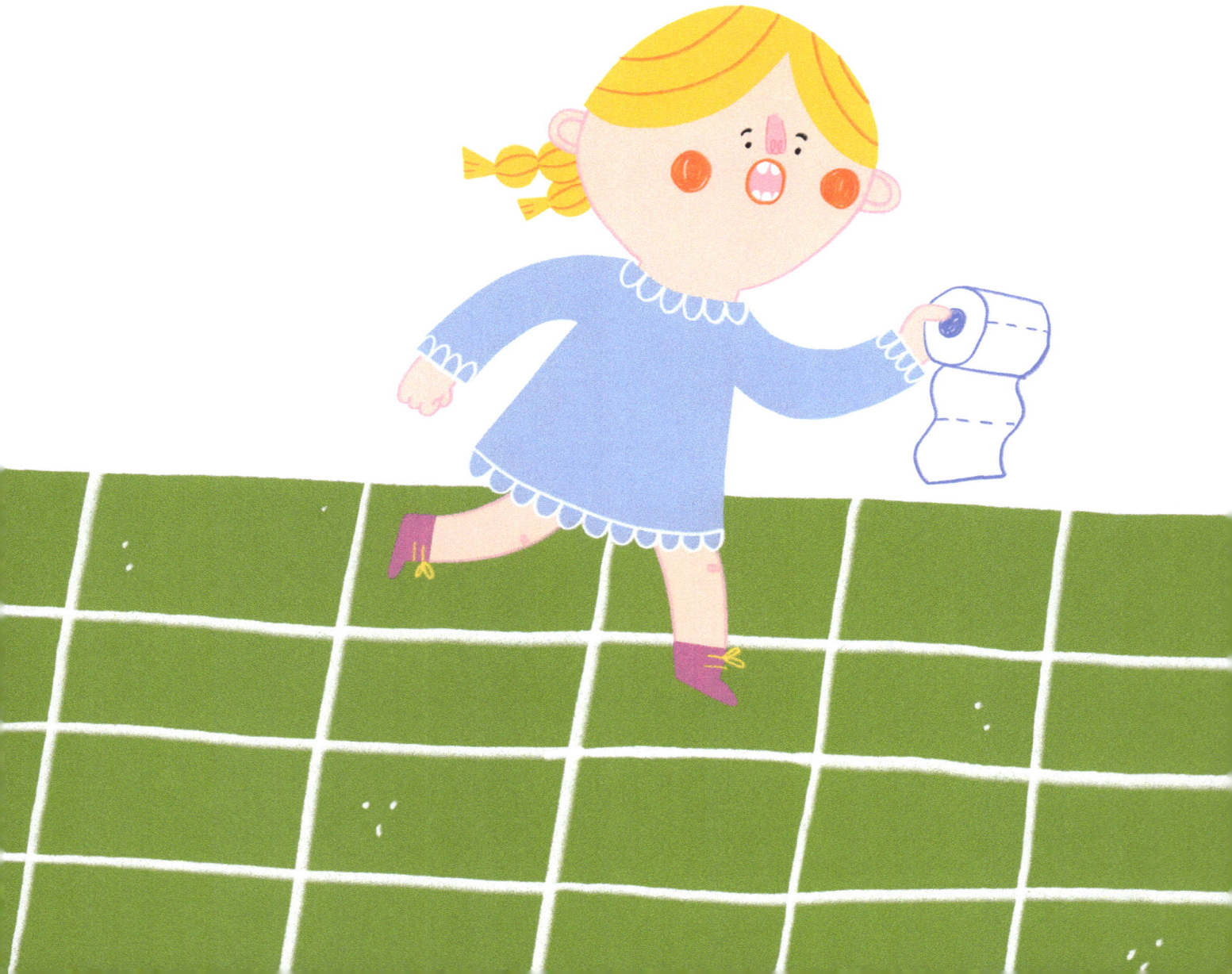

POO!

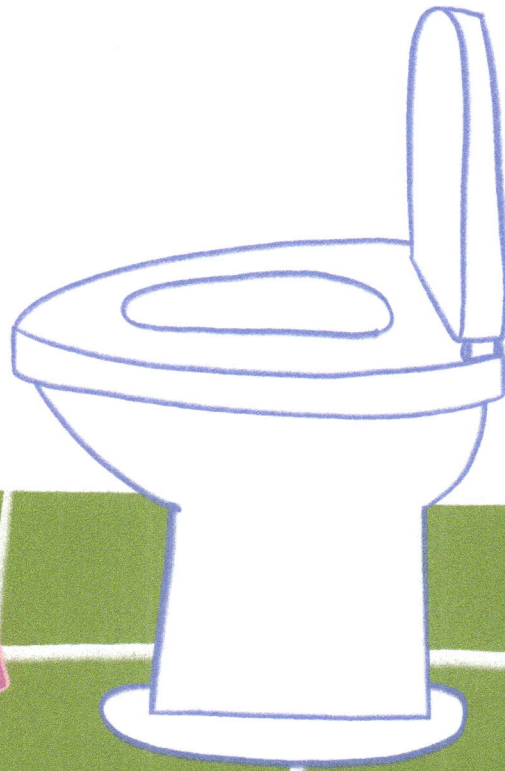
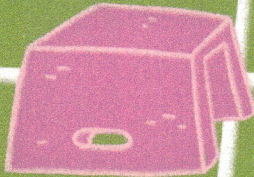

NOTES

for parents / grandparents / caregivers

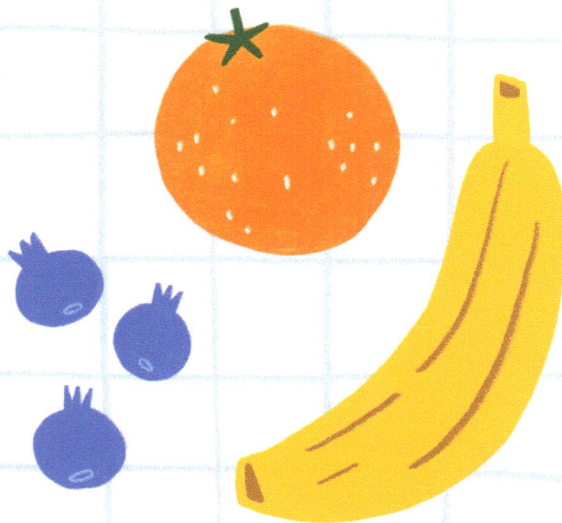

*Many of these foods contain a multitude of benefits which extend beyond the discussed organ and/or body function.

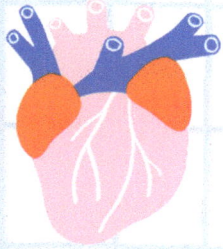

OATS contain a type of soluble fibre called beta-glucan which lowers blood glucose and cholesterol levels, thus helping to reduce the risk of heart disease and diabetes.

SALMON is rich in omega-3 fatty acids and potassium which help to reduce artery inflammation, lower cholesterol levels, and reduce the risk of heart disease.

SPINACH is a nutritional powerhouse packed with vitamins, minerals and fibre. It is particularly high in potassium and magnesium which help to relax blood vessels and lower blood pressure.

BLUEBERRIES are nutrient-dense and high in antioxidants and anthocyanidins which are believed to stimulate the flow of blood and oxygen to the brain and promote cognition and vascular health.

NUTS contain fatty acids, protein, vitamins, minerals and antioxidants which each play essential roles in many aspects of brain health including cognitive function, enhanced memory, learning and attention capacity.

AVOCADOS are full of essential nutrients and minerals which are required for brain growth and development, cell communication, cognition and psychological and neurological function.

BEETROOT and beet greens (the leaves) are rich in nitrates which have been shown to benefit lung function and optimise oxygen intake.

PUMPKINS are especially rich in carotenoids which are associated with better lung function and have powerful antioxidant and anti-inflammatory properties.

LENTILS are part of the legume family and are high in nutrients that support lung function including magnesium, iron and potassium.

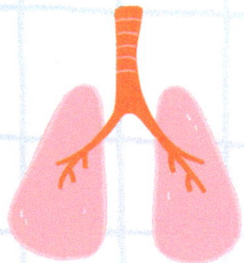

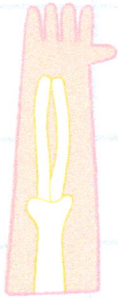

CHEESE is an excellent source of calcium and vitamin D, both essential for bone health. Adequate levels of calcium are also important for our teeth, heart, nerves, and muscles to function.

MILK is an excellent source of calcium, phosphorus and protein which are all important for bone health.

BROCCOLI is a good source of vitamin K and calcium, two vital nutrients for maintaining strong, healthy bones.

EGGS are rich in high-quality protein – supplying all 9 essential amino acids – and are therefore ideal for supporting muscle development, growth and repair.

Red **MEAT** is an excellent source of protein, iron and zinc which are essential for muscle health, development and function. White meat is also a great source of lean protein which supports muscle growth and repair.

Part of the legume family, **BEANS** are rich in fibre and non-animal protein which help to keep us satisfied and build lean muscle mass.

CARROTS contain beta-carotene, a substance that the body converts to vitamin A which is an important nutrient for eye health.

PEAS contain the carotenoids lutein and zeaxanthin which can help to protect our eyes from chronic diseases such as cataracts and age-related macular degeneration.

Citrus fruits like **ORANGES**, lemons and grapefruit are high in vitamin C which supports the health of blood vessels in the eyes.

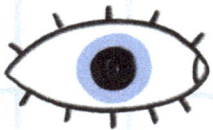

TOMATOES are an excellent source of vitamin C which can help stimulate collagen production and improve skin elasticity.

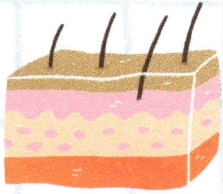

GRAPES contain an abundance of vitamin K, a nutrient which plays a critical role in blood clotting. Grapes are also high in enzymes which have anti-inflammatory effects and reparative functions for skin.

SWEET POTATOES are an excellent source of vitamin C which can help to boost collagen production which plays a role in skin elasticity and strength.

Chewing an **APPLE** stimulates saliva production which helps to rinse food particles and bacteria away from our teeth. Additionally, the vitamins and minerals found in apples such as vitamin C and potassium, contribute to gum health.

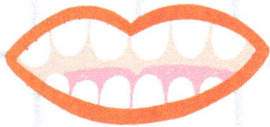

KIWI FRUITS contain high levels of vitamin C which strengthens gums and helps protect against gum inflammation called gingivitis. Kiwis are also packed full of calcium which helps to neutralise acids while boosting enamel health.

Acids from plaque, food, and other drinks can harm our tooth enamel and attract cavity-causing bacteria. Drinking **WATER** dilutes these acids, helping to fight against cavities, gum disease and protect tooth enamel.

YOGURT that is high in protein, calcium, vitamins, live cultures and probiotics can enhance gut health and digestion.

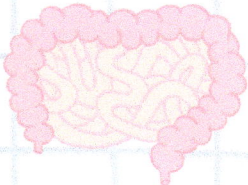

The dietary fibre in **ASPARAGUS** promotes good bacteria which helps our stomach and intestines to digest our food and absorb important nutrients.

BANANAS are high in a type of soluble fibre called pectin, which helps with digestion through regulating bowel movements and supporting the growth of good bacteria in the digestive tract.

www.ingramcontent.com/pod-product-compliance
Lightning Source LLC
Chambersburg PA
CBHW040836300326

41914CB00061B/1428